Enhancing Clinical Judgment in Nursing Practice

The art of Debriefing in Nursing

Tabassum Wazir
Bushra Sultan
Shumaila Batool

Enhancing Clinical Judgment in Nursing Practice

The art of Debriefing in Nursing

ELIVA PRESS

ISBN: 978-99993-4-207-0

Cover Design: Eliva Press
Cover Image: www.ingimage.com
Email: info@elivapress.com
Website: www.elivapress.com

This Eliva Press imprint is published by the registered company Eliva Press Global Ltd. part of Eliva Press S.R.L. Publishing Group

The registered company address is: Pope Hennessy Street Level 2, Hennessy Tower Port Louis, Mauritius
Eliva Press S.R.L. Publishing Group legal address is: Bd. Cuza-Voda 1/4 of. 21, Chisinau, Moldova, Europe

Effects of Debriefing on Clinical Judgment among Second-Year Nursing Students

Table of Contents

Chapter One: Introduction

Debriefing is a structured process involving reflective discussions between participants to review real or simulated events, helping them process emotions, analyze skills, and enhance their future performance (Palaganas et al., 2016). It enables participants to examine, evaluate, and integrate their feelings, mental processes, and other elements in a real or simulated environment to enhance their performance in real-life circumstances (Coutinho et al., 2016a; Dufrene & Young, 2014). Additionally, using debriefing as an educational intervention provides a safe environment in which students can openly analyze their clinical experiences. A key element of debriefing is reflection, which helps students articulate their learning and identify actions that could improve patient outcomes (Lavoie et al., 2017). Through critical examination, it improves clinical judgment and problem-solving abilities, and enhances self-assurance (Yun & Kang, 2022).

Moreover, as an innovative strategy, it can facilitate the development of clinical judgment abilities (Lavoie et al., 2019). It encourages students to critically assess their actions, identify mistakes, and explore alternatives, thereby enhancing their decision making and improving patient care (Guerrero et al., 2022). It helps bridge the gap between theory and practice, offers students the opportunity to reflect on their actions, receive feedback, and connect with real clinical situations (Shea, 2015). Similarly, debriefing with good judgment using the advocacy inquiry approach encourages instructors to provide clear feedback while fostering reflection from the trainees. By sharing their observations and prompting open discussions, instructors help trainees explore their decision making and improve clinical judgment (Maestre & Rudolph, 2015a). A good judgment approach promotes open dialogue through a positive approach. The 'good judgment' model encourages open discussion of mistakes, focusing on the perspectives of both instructors and trainees to promote mutual learning.

This creates space for reflection and improvement, which is crucial for enhancing patient safety (Maestre & Rudolph, 2015; Morse, 2013).

Clinical judgment is a critical aspect of nursing practice and plays a key role in ensuring patient safety and the overall quality of care. It is defined as the process of making descriptions or opinions regarding a patient's needs, concerns, or health issues and deciding whether to act, use, or alter standard methods or create new approaches based on the patient's reaction (Tanner, 2006). Clinical judgment in nursing is crucial to ensure high-quality and safe patient care (Manetti, 2018; Nielsen et al., 2016). Furthermore, it is crucial for effective decision making and is acknowledged globally as a required standard in nursing practice. (Hensel & Billings, 2020; Manetti, 2019).

Similarly, in nursing education, clinical judgment is necessary as it forms the basis for professional practice. By fostering these skills early in their training through debriefing, students learn to think critically and make informed decisions in real-life situations, thereby gradually developing the competencies necessary for effective patient care (Høegh-Larsen et al., 2023). Clinical judgment is a fundamental skill that is required by nearly all health professionals. Effective clinical judgment enhances patient outcomes by ensuring timely care, boosts safety by identifying risks, supports professional growth, and improves the quality of care through tailored, patient-centered approaches (Manetti, 2019; Victor-Chmil, 2013).

Moreover, the development of clinical judgment requires nurses to intellectually assess a patient's situation by integrating clinical reasoning and the ability to apply knowledge, as well as intuition, to inform subsequent decision-making (Manetti, 2018) . This includes understanding the patient's information, identifying deviations, making appropriate decisions, and intervening in actions. It is a multidimensional process that involves noticing, interpreting, responding, and reflecting (Yang et al., 2019).

Furthermore, clinical judgment is important to ensure safe patient-centered care in the clinical setting. It allows nurses to prioritize care, make quick decisions, manage risks, and adjust to deteriorating patient conditions (Victor-Chmil, 2013). The quality of patient care is closely linked to nurses' clinical judgment. This leads to timely interventions, reduced errors, and enhanced patient safety. It helps anticipate potential complications, thereby improving overall care standards (Okada & Tomari, 2017).

Clinical judgment is a key outcome of debriefing, particularly in nursing education and in clinical practice. Debriefing creates an opportunity for reflective learning, in which nurses and students can critically analyze their actions, thought processes, and decision-making in clinical scenarios (Høegh-Larsen et al., 2023).

To sum up, debriefing serves as a valuable approach to help nursing students strengthen their clinical judgment. Encouraging thoughtful reflection and offering constructive feedback helps students connect what they learn in the classroom with real-life practice (Cantrell et al., 2017). This process builds confidence and decision-making skills, allowing them to respond more effectively to patients' needs. When integrated into nursing education, debriefing equips students with tools they need to make informed decisions in clinical settings, ultimately leading to better patient outcomes (Sawyer et al., 2016).

Problem Statement

It has been observed as a nursing instructor, as well as a preceptee in clinical education course, that students often focus more on completing manuals than on engaging in patient care, leading to a lack of confidence and hesitation in decision-making. Students rarely have the opportunity to reflect on their performance after tasks, which limits their ability to develop clinical judgment. Post-conference discussions lack depth, hindering reflection and assessment. This approach limits the development of strong clinical judgment skills essential for competent nursing practice (Victor-Chmil, 2013). Teaching and learning strategies such as debriefing are currently being employed to address this educational gap. Understanding debriefing methods helps educators and healthcare institutions enhance their clinical judgment, leading to better practice and positive learning experiences. Although clinical judgment is a crucial academic prerequisite in nursing practice, there is an understandable lack of clinical insight and abilities among nursing trainees (Ibrahim & Aly, 2018). Moreover, another study identified that new nurse graduates frequently lack strong clinical judgment, increasing the risk of errors in patient care. Developing these skills during education is essential for safe practice (Kavanagh & Szweda, 2017).

Post-event debriefing is often overlooked by educators due to their own workload, students' tight schedules, and other curriculum demands. Evidence showing its impact on improving clinical judgment could encourage greater focus on debriefing in simulated learning (Dubula, 2018).

Significance of Study

Clinical judgment is a critical component of nursing and essential for delivering high-quality and safe patient care. Recent research underscores the importance of developing early clinical judgment in nursing education to prepare students for the complexities of real-world clinical environments (Høegh-Larsen et al., 2023; Khan et al., 2021). Similarly, the literature highlights the challenges faced by nursing students in developing clinical judgment, particularly due to the limited opportunities for reflection and critical analysis during their training (Jessee & Tanner, 2016; Lavoie et al., 2015). By enhancing students' ability to reflect on their actions, receive constructive feedback, and improve their decision-making skills, debriefing can lead to better-prepared graduates being capable of delivering safe, high-quality patient care (Palaganas et al., 2016).

This study addressed the critical aspects of nursing education and clinical practice, offering insights into effective debriefing strategies that enhance clinical judgment. These findings have the potential to improve educational outcomes, advance clinical competence, ensure patient safety, and contribute to evidence-based practice in nursing education.

Purpose

This study aimed to assess the effects of debriefing on clinical judgment among second-year nursing students.

Objectives

To assess the effectiveness of debriefing in improving the clinical judgment among second year nursing students

Research Question

What were the effects of debriefing on second-year nursing students' clinical judgment scores?

Research Hypothesis

Null Hypothesis: There is no significant difference in clinical judgment before and after debriefing among second year nursing students.

Alternate Hypothesis: Second year nursing students will demonstrate a significantly enhanced clinical judgment after undergoing debriefing.

Operational Definitions

Debriefing

Debriefing is a systematic process that involves detailed discussion between teachers and students on clinical cases. This process will be carried out to incorporate the noticing, interpreting, responding, and reflecting necessary for making clinical judgments.

Clinical Judgment:

In this study, clinical judgment was operationally defined as ability measured by the Lasater Clinical Judgment Rubric (LCJR), which assesses four dimensions: noticing, interpreting, responding, and reflecting. The scores range from 11 to 44, with higher scores indicating stronger clinical judgment skills.

Chapter Two: Literature Review

Clinical Judgment

Clinical judgment (CJ) plays a critical role in nursing and serves as a foundation for providing high-quality and safe patient care. It is essential for nurses to develop strong clinical judgment skills as these abilities enable them to make informed decisions that directly impact patient outcomes (Manetti, 2018). CJ involves the capacity to notice changes in a patient's condition, interpret the significance of these changes, respond appropriately, and reflect on outcomes to improve future practices (Dehghani, 2024).

Therefore, clinical judgment is a multifaceted process that incorporates both cognitive and practical abilities (Hensel & Billings, 2020). The words "clinical judgment," "problem solving," and "decision making," are frequently used indiscriminately (Van Graan et al., 2016).

Globally, clinical judgment is considered a core competency that nurses must possess to meet the complex demands of modern healthcare environments (Nielsen et al., 2016). The early development of clinical judgment in nursing education is crucial because it prepares nurses to handle real-world scenarios with confidence and competence (Kennedy et al., 2023).

Debriefing

Debriefing is a guided strategy in which students play an active role in determining and satisfying their learning and competency deficits. This fosters comprehension and facilitates the application of learning, talent, and attitudes with the ultimate goal of safe patient care (Elarousy et al., 2019).

Framework

Structured debriefing using the Clinical Judgment Rubric has been shown to enhance nursing students' clinical judgment, communication scores, and skill performance after simulation training, thus proving to be an effective teaching strategy (Oh, 2016).Clinical judgment is a procedure of reflection and logic that considers all available information, is supported by a vast body of knowledge, and leads to the development of a clinical decision (Connor et al., 2023).

The proposed framework for this study is Tanner's model of clinical judgment, which consists of the phases of noticing, interpreting, responding, and reflecting. The debriefing procedure emphasizes reflection both before and after. This approach, initially published in 2006, is grounded in both practice and research. Chris Tanner synthesized more than 190 nursing papers on clinical judgment. The model is in line with the nursing process to effectively develop the clinical reasoning abilities that students need to acquire for practice and licensing. According to Tanner's model, students must use four clinical reasoning processes and the way a nurse thinks to arrive at the correct clinical judgment (Tanner, 2006).

Debriefing with Good Judgement Model

A variety of frameworks and models are available to support learners through debriefing and reflection. Debriefing for Meaningful Learning (DML), Structured and Supported Debriefing, Debriefing with Good Judgment, Promoting Excellence and Reflective Education in Simulation (PEARLS), and the 3D Model of Debriefing are some of these (Badowski & Wells-Beede, 2022). These models help nursing students become more adept at clinical judgment and analytical abilities (Bradley, 2019; Fegran et al., 2023a; Zigmont et al., 2011).

In this study Debriefing with Good Judgment model is incorporated, it is a strategy that promotes open exchanges of viewpoints and personal experience. It is assumed that students strive to do their best while setting high standards and fostering an engaging learning environment (Rudolph et al., 2007). It encourages an open exchange of viewpoints and personal experiences, assumes that students are trying their utmost, and holds them to the highest possible standards while fostering an engaging learning environment. This approach entails adopting a debriefing style to extract frameworks that direct therapeutic activities, combining advocacy with inquiry, and having frank communication during debriefing (Maestre & Rudolph, 2015b).

In nursing training simulations, structured debriefing methods such as video debriefing, DML, and LCJR improve learning outcomes and the quality of debriefing more effectively than unstructured verbal discussions (Lee et al., 2020). Moreover, research has found that both oral debriefing (OD) and video-assisted debriefing (VAD) enhance learners' psychomotor abilities, self-confidence, and satisfaction while also developing emotional, cognitive, and psychosocial skills (Coutinho et al., 2016b; Ostovar et al., 2018). Despite being regarded as the "gold standard," there are no statistically significant benefits of video-assisted debriefing over instructor-led debriefing. This implies that affordable approaches can be more successful (Levett-Jones & Lapkin, 2014a). Systematic debriefing significantly increased satisfaction, with instructor-led debriefing scoring higher in perceived quality than peer-led sessions. Overall, debriefing methods were found to be effective in enhancing learning satisfaction, reflection, and psychological safety in healthcare simulations (Oh, 2016; Persico, 2017; Sultan, Dhamani, Ishtiaq, et al., 2024). Additionally, debriefing promotes thorough thinking about the entire event and learning from mistakes (Vinícius et al., 2019).

Importance of Debriefing in Nursing Education

Debriefing plays an important role in nursing education, as numerous studies have highlighted it as an essential component of the simulation process employed in clinical teaching and learning in the field of nursing (Bradley, 2019; Duff et al., 2024; Reed, 2015). Additionally, it is recognized as an organized procedure that has implications for healthcare and education (Fegran et al., 2023b). Similarly, structured debriefing enhances communication, facilitates reflection, and strengthens skills through organized feedback and discussion (Coutinho et al., 2016b).

Moreover, participants analyze real or simulated events, reflecting on their actions, emotions, mental processes, and psychomotor skills to improve future performance (Palaganas et al., 2016). Regardless of the specific technique used, debriefing has a considerable impact on the development of both technical and nontechnical skills (Levett-Jones & Lapkin, 2014b).

Impact of Debriefing on Clinical Judgment

To build clinical judgment skills, students actively evaluate their cognitive, emotional, and psychomotor performance via debriefing, an organized, and supervised reflection process. As a facilitated reflective technique, debriefing emphasizes the importance of reflection in enhancing learners' ability to make clinical judgments (AL Sabei & Lasater, 2016). Each debriefing component showed a good correlation with critical thinking. Certain aspects of debriefing have a major impact on confidence, such as consideration of clinical judgment and practice, sufficient time for debriefing, and evidence-based practice (Wallace & Gill, 2019).

Using the Lasater Clinical Judgment Scale, a mixed-methods study examined how debriefing affected nursing students' clinical judgment. Although there were no statistically significant differences in the quantitative measures, qualitative data revealed that structured debriefing had a positive impact on students' clinical judgment (Mariani et al., 2013). The clinical judgment of nursing students can be enhanced by reflecting on a simulated client deteriorating event (Lavoie et al., 2017b). Nurses must prioritize tasks and make crucial decisions that affect patient care. Nurses may not yet have the experience needed for strong clinical judgment; therefore, it is important to teach and evaluate this skill to ensure safe practice (Manetti, 2018). The use of a clinical judgment rubric in the debriefing method effectively enhances clinical judgment (Oh, 2016).

In addition, providing students with structured frameworks and opportunities for reflection is essential to fully understand and effectively apply what they have learned (Johnston, 2019). Owing to the complexity of the healthcare system, nurses must make quick and precise clinical decisions. Effective debriefing after simulation exercises provides educators a chance to improve the development of clinical judgment. A systematic debriefing strategy can help students learn more about their clinical experiences and develop nursing reasoning skills (Lusk & Fater, 2013).

A significant gap exists in the research on the impact of debriefing on clinical judgment in nursing education in Pakistan, highlighting the need to consider local cultural and educational factors. Additionally, most studies emphasize simulated environments with less focus on how debriefing affects clinical judgment in real-world settings, which is crucial for translating simulated learning into actual practice.

Western studies have provided strong evidence of the benefits of debriefing, particularly in nursing education. A mixed methods study found that reflective debriefing significantly improved nursing students' ability to analyze clinical scenarios, enhancing their clinical judgment during simulations(Lavoie et al., 2017b). Another study demonstrated that structured debriefing based on Tanner's model using the LCJR significantly enhanced clinical reasoning and decision-making skills in nursing students (Oh, 2016). Levett-Jones & Lapkin (2014) conducted a systematic review that confirmed debriefing's role in fostering clinical judgment and reducing errors in simulated environments.

Furthermore, a study highlighted that debriefing is integral to simulation-based education, allowing students to reflect on their actions and improve their clinical judgment (Dreifuerst, 2015). By examining how a debriefing procedure improves students' capacity to handle challenging clinical scenarios with self-confidence and judgment, this study examines the effects of debriefing on clinical judgment in post-clinical conferences on case discussions among second-year nursing students.

Research Methodology

Study Design

This study employed a quasi-experimental design with pre- and post-tests (Gray & Grove, 2013).

Study Setting and Duration

This study was conducted at a private nursing college in Islamabad from November 2023 to October 2024. This institute offers a four-year programme. A significant component of the program is clinical practice, which provides students with hands-on experiences in various healthcare settings. This practical exposure is crucial for developing clinical skills and for understanding real-world nursing challenges. It develops students' competencies in assessing, diagnosing, and managing health problems with skills in care planning, medication administration, wound care, and patient education. It also emphasizes critical thinking and decision making in complex clinical scenarios.

Eligibility Criteria for Participants

Eligibility criteria define the characteristics needed for inclusion in the target population based on the research problem, purpose, literature, and study design (Gray & Grove, 2013). Participants who met the eligibility criteria were included in this study. The inclusion and exclusion criteria were as follows:

The inclusion criteria for the study were Bachelor of Science in Nursing (BSN) students enrolled in the Adult Health Nursing II course.

The exclusion criteria included students who were on leave for three or more days during clinical sessions as well as those who were repeating or retaking the course.

Sampling and Sample Size

Census sampling method used in this study. All participants who met the inclusion criteria were invited to participate in this study.

A well-defined group of second-year Bachelor of Science in Nursing (BSN) students enrolled in the Adult Health Nursing (AHN) II course who met the sampling criteria of the study were selected (Gray & Grove, 2013). The sample size was 53 students. Among them 70 percent students were female and 30 percent were male with in age range from 18 to 25 years. AHN II students usually have considerable practical exposure to completing basic nursing courses. Their clinical objectives involved utilization of the nursing process to provide care to adults. These students were chosen because they had completed basic nursing courses, which made them suitable for studying how debriefing affected clinical judgment. Their expected level of expertise allows researchers to effectively evaluate how debriefing could improve their clinical judgment.

Recruitment Process

Initially, permission was obtained from the Head of Department (HOD) for the recruitment of participants and training of clinical teachers involved in data collection and intervention implementation. After approval, information sheets were provided to the year coordinator to inform them about the study. With the permission of the assistant dean of undergraduate students, the program secretary was approached to acquire a list of eligible participants and faculty members who were involved in the clinical teaching of AHN II. Clinical teachers were selected for the data collection and implementation of the intervention.

Data Collection Tool

Data related to gender, age, and previous experience of debriefing were collected on the demographic data sheet. Clinical judgment was measured using the adapted Lasater Clinical Judgment Rubric (LCJR).

Instrument Lasater Clinical Judgment Rubric

This study utilized the adapted Lasater Clinical Judgment Rubric developed by Kathie Lasater (2007) to collect data. Permission to use and restate the statements in rubric format was obtained from the primary author. The LCJR assesses four main dimensions of clinical judgment: noticing, interpreting, responding, and reflecting (Lasater, 2007). It comprises 11 items distributed across these dimensions: three items for noticing, two for interpreting, four for responding, and two for reflecting. Each item is rated on a 4-point scale: exemplary (4), accomplished (3), developing (2), and beginning (1). The total scores ranged from 11 to 44. The LCJR demonstrated a reliability coefficient of .90 using Chronbach's alpha (Cantrell et al., 2021).

The Lasater Clinical Judgment Rubric (LCJR) has been widely used in various studies to assess the development of clinical judgment among nursing students through simulations and debriefing. It has proven to be a valuable tool in both educational and clinical settings, facilitating the evaluation of students' clinical judgment skills (Mariani et al., 2013; Nunes et al., 2020; Sultan, Victor, Naeem, et al., 2024; Weaver, 2015).

Data Collection Process

The adapted LCJR was utilized in two ways: self-administered and teacher-administered. In the self-administered LCJR, the students rated their clinical judgment before and after the intervention. Moreover, teacher-administered LCJR was marked by clinical teachers who marked the students' clinical judgment at the time of the first clinical case discussion in fourth and fifth week with the student to obtain baseline data. Furthermore, post data were collected on the last clinical case discussion in 11th and 12th week in post conferences.

Intervention

The intervention was organized and reported according to the TIDieR (Template for Intervention Description and Replication) checklist. This approach was used to ensure a systematic and comprehensive description of all key components of the intervention, including rationale, materials, procedures, and delivery methods (Ided, 2014).

Brief Name

Debriefing with the Good Judgment Model. This model emphasizes four key components: noticing, interpreting, responding, and reflecting, with a focus on clinical decision making and reasoning behind actions (Tanner, 2006).

Figure 2. Intervention Implementation Model

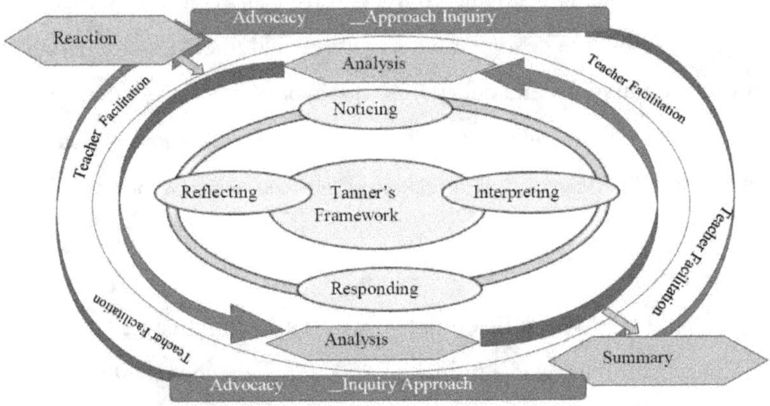

Why (Rationale for Intervention)

The intervention was implemented to enhance clinical judgment by focusing on the key components of clinical judgment (noticing, interpreting, responding, and reflecting) and facilitating reflective learning (Maestre & Rudolph, 2015b).

What (materials)

The intervention involved debriefing planners, debriefing sessions, case discussions, open-ended questions with advocacy and inquiry approaches, and a supportive environment that encouraged active participation and reflection (Coggins et al., 2021; El-gebaly et al., 2021; Kim & Son, 2022; Mariani et al., 2013).

What (procedures)

The students were divided into groups and collaboratively developed a clinical planner along with a debriefing planner to schedule debriefing sessions, ensuring at least three sessions for each student. The students participated in post-clinical debriefing sessions, discussed cases using Good Judgment, and incorporated Tanner's clinical judgment model. Debriefing with Good Judgment Model includes three phases: reaction/description, analysis, and summarization(Maestre & Rudolph, 2015b). Tanner's Framework includes noticing, interpreting, responding, and reflecting, with a focus on clinical decision-making and reasoning behind actions. They engaged in reflective discussions on clinical judgment supported by the teacher's facilitation (Maestre & Rudolph, 2015a; Modic & Schoessler, 2013; Morse, 2013). During intervention debriefing with good judgment model was utilized. In which Student explain the case in reaction phase and also express their reaction. Then they move to analysis phase which is the critical phase of debriefing. During analysis phase students were move through the tanner framework. Teachers direct the students through advocacy inquiry approach to their notification of changes & their interpretation and how they respond. Later they reflect on situation how they behave, act and what were their area of improvement in their learning. In last they summarize the case and teacher provide feedback.

Who Provided?

Trained clinical teachers conducted the debriefing sessions. Clinical teachers, who were involved in clinical rotations in the second year of AHN II, implemented debriefing during the clinical case discussion. The eligibility criterion for clinical teachers was having a post-RN or BSN degree. Moreover, they had at least six months of clinical teaching experience and a minimum of two years of clinical experience.

Clinical Teacher's Training

Clinical teachers were trained for the debriefing intervention. Moreover, the purpose of the study and a description of the tool were provided to clinical teachers. This training covered debriefing techniques and the utilization of the LCJR to ensure consistency. The debriefing training was conducted by the

Primary Investigator (PI) and an expert in two workshops during the second and third weeks of the semester. Each workshop lasted for three hours.

Workshop 1

In the first workshop, the theoretical content was covered, focusing on key topics such as the concept of debriefing, a Good Judgment model, various models of debriefing, Tanner's Clinical Judgment model, and the role of instructors in facilitating effective debriefing sessions. Additionally, the workshop included an overview of the adapted Lasater Clinical Judgment Rubric (LCJR) and explained its use as a tool for collecting and assessing data related to clinical judgment. This comprehensive coverage ensured that clinical teachers were well prepared to apply both debriefing techniques and LCJR in a consistent and informed manner during the intervention.

Workshop 2

The researcher conducted a role play of debriefing with the Good Judgment Model incorporating Tanner's clinical judgment model on a clinical scenario to demonstrate the debriefing in front of clinical teachers. Following this, two different clinical scenarios were given to clinical teachers for return demonstration. Clinical teachers were divided into two pairs; they practiced that clinical scenario and then demonstrated it in front of others. Both pairs of teachers were allowed to give feedback and comments on demonstrations to each other. The PI and expert clarified the concerns and queries and provided feedback.

How Delivered: Implementation Process

In the clinical setting, the student selected a patient, discussed them with the clinical teacher, and clarified their concerns. The teachers observed students' involvement in patient care throughout the day, noting their actions and decisions. The students were asked to discuss their cases with the clinical teacher during the debriefing session. They were given a few minutes to reflect on what went well, the areas needing improvement, and their overall approach to patient care.

To facilitate students in debriefing discussions, teachers used the following questions:

Please explain your case thoroughly.

Have you noticed any issues or problems in this case? How did you identify this issue?

Could you reflect on the situation again and tell me what could be the most appropriate way to deal with the situation?

What is your response to this case? What actions were taken to manage the case, and what will your plan for further care of this patient?

Please conclude the whole case and give your reflection on it.

What is your learning from this case and session?

What do you take from this experience in your future clinical practice?

What do you do if you have the opportunity to face the same case in the future?

Where (location)

The intervention was conducted during post-clinical conferences in a separate calm environment to promote open communication and active participation.

When & How Much

Debriefing sessions were conducted after each clinical on case discussion in the post-clinical conference. Every student had the opportunity to participate in at least three debriefing sessions. Each debriefing session was expected to last between 30 minutes (timings may vary based on discussion). The debriefing planner was shared with the clinical teachers and participants. The full implementation of the debriefing intervention commenced in the fourth week of the semester and continued through the twelfth week.

Tailoring

The intervention was tailored to the clinical experiences of each student, with the teachers adapting the discussions based on individual cases and learning needs. Teachers tailored their debriefing approach by first reviewing the student's specific clinical experience, allowing them to highlight relevant experiences, such as challenges faced during patient care. This ensured that the reflection process was grounded in the student's real-world clinical practice. The teacher's feedback was then adjusted to target areas where the student demonstrated strength or required further development (Shaub, 2019; Van Vliet et al., 2016).

Modifications

No significant modifications were reported during the implementation of the intervention (Ided, 2014).

How Well (Planned & Actual)

The fidelity of the intervention was ensured using comprehensive strategies. Clinical teachers underwent training on debriefing techniques and the Lasater Clinical Judgment Rubric (LCJR) with two workshops covering both theory and practical applications. A pilot test helped refine the debriefing process before full implementation and feedback was used to improve question clarity and session flow. Debriefing with Good Judgment Model, incorporating Tanner's Clinical Judgment Model, was consistently applied. Teachers followed a standardized set of questions during the debriefing sessions, which were recorded and sent to the Primary Investigator (PI). The PI and supervisor reviewed the recordings after a few sessions and provided feedback to ensure smooth intervention. The PI also made regular visits to observe the debriefing sessions to ensure consistency.

The debriefing sessions were held regularly, with each student participating in at least three sessions. Data were collected pre- and post-intervention using the LCJR to measure the impact on clinical judgment. These steps maintained the integrity and effectiveness of the intervention.

Data Analysis

Data were analyzed using SPSS version 26 and Microsoft Excel. The PI entered the data into the software and conducted data screening to identify and address any missing or redundant entries before the analysis. Descriptive and inferential statistics were used in this study. Normality of the data was checked using kurtosis and skewness, Shapiro-Wilk test, QQ plot, and histogram. All data were examined for accuracy. Normality was achieved; therefore, a dependent T test was applied to compare the LCJR scores.

Descriptive statistics, such as mean and frequency distributions, were used for demographic data. Inferential statistics such as paired t-test was used to compare pre- and post-intervention clinical judgment scores, which revealed significant improvements in both teacher-rated and student self-rated scores. Each dimension of the Lasater Clinical Judgment Rubric (LCJR) was analyzed separately to determine the impact of debriefing on specific aspects of clinical judgment. A detailed item-level analysis of the LCJR was conducted to explore changes in the frequency and percentage of participants across different performance levels.

Ethical Consideration

Ethical approval was obtained from the Institutional Review Board and Ethical Committee of Shifa Tameer-e-Millat University (reference #061-24)). Permission was granted using the Lasater Clinical Judgment Rubric (LCJR) scale. Furthermore, permission was obtained from the dean of the College of Nursing for data collection from the participants and conducting a workshop for trainers. The purpose of this study was shared with all participants. Autonomy was ensured by obtaining informed consent from each participant who was allowed to withdraw from the study at any time. Written consent was obtained from the clinical teachers. Participants were also given the opportunity to ask any question related to the study. Confidentiality was maintained by hiding their name and ID's and giving a serial code instead. Codes were used for each participant to maintain anonymity. All participants were exposed to the intervention as they were likely to provide valuable benefits. This approach ensured fairness and alignment with the principle of beneficence, promoting equal opportunities for all participants to improve their clinical judgment skills. In doing so, the study upheld ethical standards by maximizing potential positive outcomes for everyone involved. Multiple debriefing sessions with each participant enhanced the improvement in clinical judgment, sensitized them, and reduced their fear of low marking by the teacher. All the information obtained from the participants was highly confidential. All raw data were kept in a lock and key, and soft data were secured with password protection on a personal computer. Nobody had accessed the information, except for the PI and the thesis committee.

Results

Demographic Characteristics of Participants

The mean age of the 53 participants was 20.5 (SD = 1.76) years, with an age range of 18 to 25 years (Table 1). The majority (74%) of the participants were between 18 and 21 years old. Moreover, in terms of gender, the majority (70%) of the participants were female.

Table 1

Demographic Characteristics of the Participants (n = 53)

Characteristics	Frequencies	(%)
Age		20.5±1.76*
18-21	39	74
22-25	14	26

Gender		
Male	16	30
Female	37	70

***Mean** ± SD

Comparison of Overall Scores of Clinical Judgment

The overall results of clinical judgment scores indicated significant improvements in both teacher-rated and student self-rated scores from pre- to post-intervention (Table 2).

For teacher-rated scores, the post-intervention means score of 35.77(SD = 5.65) was higher than the pre-intervention mean score of 15.42 (SD = 2.25), with a statistically significant p-value ($p < 0.001$).

Similarly, for student self-rated scores, the post-intervention mean score of 38.08 (SD = 4.06) was higher than the pre-intervention mean score of 12.25 (SD = 0.92), with a statistically significant p-value ($p < 0.001$). Moreover, in post-intervention, the students' self-rated mean scores of 38.08 (SD= 4.06) were higher than the teacher-rated mean scores of 35.77 (SD=5.65). Overall, the students rated themselves higher than the teacher, as evidenced by their mean scores. Moreover, Cohen's d values (Teacher-rated = 3.46, student self-rated = 5.35) indicated a large effect size of the intervention.

Table 2

Overall Comparison of Clinical Judgment Scores

	Pre-Intervention		**Post-Intervention**		**t-value**	**df$^{\$}$**	**p-value**
	Mean	±SD$^{\#}$	Mean	±SD$^{\#}$			
Teacher' s rated scores	15.4	2.25	35.77	5.65	-25.20	52	0.001
Student's self-rated scores	12.25	0.92	38.08	4.06	-46.25	52	0.001
Cohen's d: Teacher' s rated = 3.46, Student's self-rated = 5.35							

SD$^{\#}$ = Standard Deviation, df$^{\$}$ = Degrees of Freedom.

Comparison of Clinical Judgment Scores for Each Item

Debriefing significantly enhanced clinical judgment abilities among second-year nursing students across all the dimensions. The analysis of each dimension of the clinical judgment rubric showed significant differences between the pre- and post-intervention scores (Table 3). The mean differences before and after debriefing were statistically significant in all dimensions: noticing, interpreting, responding, and reflecting for both teachers' and students' self-rated scores (mentioned above).

For teacher-rated scores, the mean scores in each dimension improved post-intervention, such as effective noticing post scores mean 9.98 (SD = 2.67), in comparison to pre 3.60 (SD = 0.32), effective interpreting post scores mean 6.34 (SD = 1.50), as compared to pre 2.28 (SD = 0.25), responding post scores mean was12.92 (SD = 4.42), pre scores 5.96 (SD = 3.00), and in reflecting post scores mean was 6.53 (SD = 1.52) in comparison to pre-intervention scores 3.57 (SD = 0.48]). Moreover, there was a statistically significant difference, with p-values less than 0.001 in each dimension.

For student self-rated scores, the mean score in each dimension was improved post-intervention; therefore, noticing mean scores were 10.58 (SD = 1.67) as compared to the pre-intervention mean of 3.38 (SD = 0.28). Effective interpreting post-intervention mean scores of 6.70 (SD = 1.14) increased from a pre-intervention mean of 2.21 (SD = 0.17), in responding a post-intervention mean of 14.06 (SD = 2.09) as compared to pre-intervention mean of 4.42 (SD = 0.40). Effective reflecting, post-intervention mean of 6.74 (SD = 1.12) in comparison with pre-intervention mean of 2.25 (SD = 0.19. Additionally, there was a statistically significant difference, with p-values less than 0.001 in each dimension.

The post-intervention mean scores of students self-rated in all dimensions of clinical judgment were higher than the post-intervention mean scores of the teachers. The results in Table 3 showed a statistically significant difference in mean scores, with higher post-intervention scores compared to pre-intervention scores ($p < 0.05$). This indicates an improvement in students' clinical judgment following the debriefing sessions.

Based on this, the Null Hypothesis is rejected, and the Alternate Hypothesis: Second-year nursing students will demonstrate significantly enhanced clinical judgment after undergoing debriefing, is supported by the findings.

Table 3

Comparison of Scores in Each Dimensions of Clinical Judgment

Dimensions	Pre-Intervention		Post-Intervention		t-value	df$	P-value
	Mean	±SD#	Mean	±SD#			
Teacher's rated scores							
Effective Noticing	3.6	0.32	9.98	2.67	-28.25	52	0.001
Effective Interpreting	2.28	0.25	6.34	1.5	-21.87	52	0.001
Effective Responding	5.96	3	12.92	4.42	-20.25	52	0.001
Effective Reflecting	3.57	0.48	6.53	1.52	-14.97	52	0.001
Student's self-rated scores							
Effective Noticing	3.38	0.28	10.58	1.67	-34.73	52	0.001
Effective Interpreting	2.21	0.17	6.7	1.14	-29.19	52	0.001
Effective Responding	4.42	0.4	14.06	2.09	-47.37	52	0.001
Effective Reflecting	2.25	0.19	6.74	1.12	-28.33	52	0.001

SD# = Standard Deviation, df$ = Degrees of Freedom.

Chapter Five: Discussion

The study findings revealed a significant improvement in the clinical judgment scores of second-year nursing students following the debriefing intervention, with a Good Judgment Model incorporating Tanner's clinical judgment model, thus rejecting the null hypothesis. These findings suggest that debriefing as a teaching strategy is effective in enhancing clinical judgment skills among second-year nursing students. These findings are consistent with those of previous studies (Byrne et al., 2023; Oh, 2016). Oh (2016) reported that structured debriefing using a clinical judgment rubric significantly enhances clinical judgment and communication. Similarly, Byrne et al. (2023) found that structured debriefing significantly improves nursing students' clinical judgment, critical thinking, and self-reflection, especially in managing long-term health conditions. Furthermore, these findings also align with research demonstrating that structured reflective debriefing improves nursing students' clinical judgment in simulations of patient deterioration, highlighting the effectiveness of a systematic review approach and assessment during debriefing. This process reinforces observational and interpretation skills, which are crucial components of clinical judgment (Lavoie et al., 2017b). However, in contrast, Shaub (2019) reviewed the evidence on the use of structured debriefing in simulation-based learning (SBL) for nursing students and found that quantitative data did not consistently demonstrate statistically significant improvements in clinical judgment after debriefing sessions(Shaub, 2019).

Interestingly, in the current study, the students' self-rated scores were higher than teacher-rated scores, suggesting that students perceived a more significant improvement in their clinical judgment than teachers did. This is likely due to the reflective nature of debriefing with the Good Judgment Model using the advocacy inquiry approach, which fosters an environment in which students critically evaluate their decisions and actions in a clinical setting. This approach promotes self-assessment and provides insights into complex scenarios (Farrington et al., 2019). Similarly, previous studies have found that self-reflection offers students valuable insights that enhance their clinical judgment (Morse, 2013; Sultan, Victor, & Begum Gul, 2024). As Sultan et al.(2024) explained, reflection involves the ability to critically evaluate one's own experiences, thoughts, and actions, making it a vital component of clinical judgment and critical thinking in nursing practice. Morse (2013) also noted that reflection is a critical component of the learning process, particularly when using the Debriefing with Good Judgment model incorporating Tanner's Clinical Judgment model, which involves a deep exploration of the internal frames of reference or mental models that guide clinical behaviors and decision-making.

Similarly, in terms of age, this is the stage of development where the participants are transitioning from adolescence into early adulthood, a period marked by increased self-awareness and growing confidence in their abilities. Previous research suggests that reflection tends to deepen with age, as individuals develop greater self-awareness and the ability to critically examine their actions and decisions (Bulman, 2013).

In the domain of effective noticing, two items showed significant differences between teacher-rated and student self-rated scores: recognizing deviations from expected patterns, and focused observation. For the focused observation item, both students and teachers acknowledged a substantial improvement in their ability to observe critical patient cues after the intervention. However, for the item recognizing deviation from expected patterns, there was a significant difference, with students rating themselves higher than the teacher ratings.

This discrepancy may be attributed to the effects of the debriefing intervention, which likely enhanced the students' confidence in their ability to recognize deviations in patient conditions. These findings align with those of previous studies (Ayed et al., 2022; Dreifuerst, 2015). According to Ayed et al. (2022), a key factor in the success of high-fidelity simulations is the debriefing process, which plays a critical role in the development of clinical judgment. Debriefing allows nursing students to reflect on their experiences, thus bridging the gap between theory and practice. It significantly improved the students' ability to identify critical clinical cues, demonstrating the effectiveness of the intervention in developing this essential aspect of clinical judgment. Dreifuerst (2015), indicated that debriefing helps nursing students become more attentive to patient cues, leading to better clinical judgment and learning. This indicates that debriefing may help reinforce observational skills that are fundamental in clinical practice.

Moreover, the present study demonstrated that in the domain of effective interpreting, both prioritizing data and making sense of data showed marked improvement after debriefing and significant differences between teacher-rated and student self-rated scores. Second-year nursing students rated themselves as slightly higher. The debriefing process enables second-year nursing students to make sense of the clinical information they notice and prioritize it according to the different conditions of the patient to participate in the patient's clinical decision for further planning. These results are consistent with those of previous studies (Dubula, 2018; Kawase et al., 2024). As Dubula (2018) indicated, debriefing enhances the ability to interpret clinical data more effectively, promoting better decision-making. Similarly, Kawase et al., (2024) found that through simulation debriefing, participants learned the importance of gathering information, interpreting the findings, and anticipating future events based on current conditions. These findings are consistent with (Yang et al., 2019), who demonstrated improved ability in nursing students to recognize changes in their patients' conditions, as well as enhanced skills in seeking information, interpreting, prioritizing, and making sense of data.

Additionally, in the domain of effective responding, the debriefing process significantly improved students' preparedness and ability to respond to clinical situations in a calm and confident manner. The intervention enabled second-year students to actively reflect on clinical data, prioritize their actions, and develop more effective response strategies during clinical practice. These findings are similar to those of a previous study showing a notable statistical difference between the scores before and after debriefing, indicating enhanced skills in communication, flexibility, and confidence during patient care (Dubula, 2018).

Students rated themselves highly confident and able to respond calmly and effectively after the debriefing sessions, indicating a strong sense of self-awareness. In contrast, teachers rated, while acknowledging the improvement, slightly lower scores indicated cautious assessment, considering the criticality of this aspect in a clinical setting. This difference suggests that the students found themselves more confident, while the teachers found it with gradual progression, highlighting the need for more support from teachers in this particular aspect in the future. A previous study supported these findings; while students often feel more confident after training, instructors tend to assess them more cautiously, recognizing the complexities of real-world practice that students may not yet fully grasp (McCabe et al., 2016).

For well-planned intervention/flexibility, contrary results were obtained, with teachers rating students more highly than students rated themselves. This suggests that, while students were still building confidence in planning and adjusting interventions, teachers recognized a more noticeable improvement in their critical thinking and adaptability. This is consistent with a study in which The Lasater Clinical Judgment Rubric (LCJR) was utilized to assess nursing students' clinical reasoning abilities during simulated patient care scenarios. Both nursing students and faculty participated in completing the tool; faculty rated students higher in the responding and reflecting dimensions, whereas students self-rated higher in other dimensions (Jensen, 2013).

Finally, in the domain of effective reflection, debriefing substantially enhanced students' ability to reflect on their clinical practice, an essential component of ongoing learning. The structured debriefing approach with the Good Judgment Model may have allowed learners to engage in meaningful self-reflection, leading to enhanced clinical judgment and critical thinking over time. Through facilitated discussions and focused feedback, the participants were better able to identify the strengths and areas that needed improvement. This is consistent with a previous study that showed significant improvement after the intervention. Deeper reflection from Debriefing with Good Judgment may have driven the sustained high level of reflection (Dubula, 2018; Morse, 2013). In this domain, both evaluation/self-analysis and commitment to improvement items demonstrated differences between teacher-rated and self-rated scores. For evaluation/self-analysis, both students and teachers rated participants equally at the accomplished level, indicating consensus on the progress made in students' ability to reflect on their clinical performance. Moreover, Debriefing with Good Judgment model and Tanner's clinical judgment framework could promote reflection. Factors such as the situation modality, experience level, and instructional strategies may also play a role in enhancing reflective ability, highlighting the complexity of reflective learning. According to a previous study, debriefing can be viewed as students' process of acquiring new insights into their professional development. This process is reflected in three key areas: enhancing the ability to provide and receive feedback, readiness for action, and progress through self-discovery (Husebø et al., 2024).

This close alignment may be due to the emphasis placed on self-reflection during the debriefing sessions, where second-year nursing students were encouraged to critically assess their decision-making processes. As noted by Mariani (2013), structured reflection during debriefing enhances students' ability to objectively evaluate their clinical actions, which could explain why teachers and students rate this item similarly.

Teachers rated the students at an exemplary level of commitment to improvement, which suggests that they observed a strong commitment from students to continually improve their clinical judgment. However, second-year nursing students may still feel that they have areas to work on, possibly due to the self-awareness gained through reflective debriefing. As students become more aware of their limitations, they may rate themselves more critically, as they strive to meet the high standards set by their instructors. In support of these findings, previous research has found that nursing students indicated that reflective debriefing improves their self-evaluation and reflection skills. It helped them recall what they had learned, identify their strengths and weaknesses, express their thoughts, and analyze their performance. They also became more independent in mastering skills, enhanced their observations, and gained new ways of thinking through reflection (El-gebaly et al., 2021). These are in contrast with Jensen (2013), in which students rated themselves slightly higher than faculty.

Limitation of Study

This study was conducted in one setting, which may limit the generalizability of the findings to a larger population. Individual differences in teaching styles could be a limitation and may have influenced the intervention, even though all the teachers underwent the training. The findings may primarily apply to second-year nursing students, limiting the generalizability to older or more experienced students. Most of the existing literature focuses on high-fidelity simulations rather than actual clinical settings, which might limit comparisons and contextual applicability.

Strengths of Study

The clinical debriefing intervention, using the debriefing with a Good Judgment model, was clearly defined and implemented systematically, providing a targeted approach to enhancing clinical judgment. One of the key strengths of this study was the teacher's training in the implementation of the intervention. Moreover, the comprehensive assessment approach further strengthened this study. Incorporating both teacher evaluations and student self-assessments provides a well-rounded perspective on students' clinical judgment skills. The use of robust statistical methods, including effect size calculations, further strengthens the credibility of the results, ensuring that the findings are both reliable and meaningful. Additionally, the study's use of the Lasater Clinical Judgment Rubric (LCJR) adds validity to the assessment as it is a widely accepted tool for measuring clinical judgment in nursing education.

Implications and Recommendations

In Nursing Education:

The study emphasizes integrating structured debriefing, such as the Debriefing with Good Judgment model, into curricula to enhance clinical judgment, reflection, and decision-making. It also highlights the need for standardized training of clinical instructors to ensure effective and consistent debriefing practices.

In Clinical Settings:

Debriefing improves clinical judgment, leading to better decision-making, reduced errors, and enhanced patient safety. It also promotes reflective practice and continuous professional growth in real-world care.

In Future Research:

Further studies should explore the long-term effects of debriefing, use control or randomized designs, and include diverse populations to strengthen evidence and generalizability.

Conclusion

This study demonstrates that the Good Judgment Model of debriefing effectively enhances second-year nursing students' clinical judgment, particularly in observation, reflection, interpretation, and response. Despite some variation in the literature, the findings support integrating structured debriefing into nursing education to improve decision-making and patient care. The results also have implications for clinical practice and patient safety, with further research needed to refine debriefing strategies and strengthen outcomes.

References

AL Sabei, S. D., & Lasater, K. (2016). Simulation debriefing for clinical judgment development: A concept analysis. *Nurse Education Today*, *45*, 42–47. https://doi.org/10.1016/j.nedt.2016.06.008

Ayed, A., Khalaf, I. A., Fashafsheh, I., Saleh, A., Bawadi, H., Abuidhail, J., Thultheen, I., & Joudallah, H. (2022). Effect of High-Fidelity Simulation on Clinical Judgment Among Nursing Students. *Inquiry (United States)*, *59*, 1–6. https://doi.org/10.1177/00469580221081997

Badowski, D., & Wells-Beede, E. (2022). State of Prebriefing and Debriefing in Virtual Simulation. *Clinical Simulation in Nursing*, *62*, 42–51. https://doi.org/10.1016/j.ecns.2021.10.006

Bradley, C. S. (2019). Impact of Training on Use of Debriefing for Meaningful Learning. *Clinical Simulation in Nursing*, *32*, 13–19. https://doi.org/10.1016/j.ecns.2019.04.003

Bulman, C. (2013). An Introduction to Reflection. In *Reflective Practice in Nursing*. https://doi.org/10.2307/466183

Byrne, D., Blumenfeld, S., Szulewski, M., & Laske, R. A. (2023). Using Simulation to Develop Clinical Judgment in Undergraduate Nursing Students. *Home Healthcare Now*, *41*(2), 84–89. https://doi.org/10.1097/NHH.0000000000001143

Cantrell, M. A., Franklin, A., Leighton, K., & Carlson, A. (2017). The Evidence in Simulation-Based Learning Experiences in Nursing Education and Practice: An Umbrella Review. *Clinical Simulation in Nursing*, *13*(12), 634–667. https://doi.org/10.1016/j.ecns.2017.08.004

Cantrell, M. A., Mariani, B., & Lengetti, E. (2021). Internal Reliability Estimates of the Lasater Clinical Judgment Rubric Among New-to-Practice Nurses in a Simulated Setting. *Nursing Education Perspectives*, *42*(6), E49–E51. https://doi.org/10.1097/01.NEP.0000000000000802

Coggins, A., Zaklama, R., Szabo, R. A., Diaz-Navarro, C., Scalese, R. J., Krogh, K., & Eppich, W. (2021). Twelve tips for facilitating and implementing clinical debriefing programmes. *Medical Teacher*, *43*(5), 509–517. https://doi.org/10.1080/0142159X.2020.1817349

Connor, J., Flenady, T., Massey, D., & Dwyer, T. (2023). Clinical judgement in nursing – An evolutionary concept analysis. *Journal of Clinical Nursing*, *32*(13–14), 3328–3340. https://doi.org/10.1111/jocn.16469

Coutinho, V. R. D., Martins, J. C. A., & Pereira, F. (2016a). Structured debriefing in nursing simulation: students' perceptions. *Journal of Nursing Education and Practice*, *6*(9), 127–134. https://doi.org/10.5430/jnep.v6n9p127

Coutinho, V. R. D., Martins, J. C. A., & Pereira, F. (2016b). Structured debriefing in nursing simulation: students' perceptions. *Journal of Nursing Education and Practice*, *6*(9), 127–134. https://doi.org/10.5430/jnep.v6n9p127

Dehghani, A. (2024). Development and validation of the clinical judgment capability questionnaire in nurses: A sequential exploratory mixed method study. *International Journal of Nursing Studies Advances*, *6*(March), 100191. https://doi.org/10.1016/j.ijnsa.2024.100191

Dreifuerst, K. T. (2015). Getting started with debriefing for meaningful learning. *Clinical Simulation in Nursing*, *11*(5), 268–275. https://doi.org/10.1016/j.ecns.2015.01.005

Dubula, M. (2018). Simulation Debriefing and the Development of Clinical Judgement of Student Nurses at a University in Gauteng. *Advancing the Science of Healthcare Simulation June 13-16, 2018, Toronto, Canada*, *7*, 1–25.

Duff, J. P., Morse, K. J., Seelandt, J., Gross, I. T., Lydston, M., Sargeant, J., Dieckmann, P., Allen, J. A., Rudolph, J. W., & Kolbe, M. (2024). Debriefing Methods for Simulation in Healthcare: A Systematic Review. *Simulation in Healthcare*, *19*(1), S112–S121. https://doi.org/10.1097/SIH.0000000000000765

Dufrene, C., & Young, A. (2014). Successful debriefing - Best methods to achieve positive learning outcomes: A literature review. *Nurse Education Today*, *34*(3), 372–376. https://doi.org/10.1016/j.nedt.2013.06.026

Elarousy, W., Beer, J. de, & Alnajjar, H. (2019). Exploring the Experiences of Nursing Students during Debriefing: A Qualitative Study. *American Journal of Nursing Research*, *7*(3), 310–315. https://doi.org/10.12691/ajnr-7-3-11

El-gebaly, S. M., El-Hawashy, Z. I., AbouShosha, A. E. F., & Abdel Haleim, G. E. (2021). The Effectiveness of Reflective Debriefing Strategy in Nursing Education. *International Journal of Novel Research in Healthcare and Nursing*, *8*(1), 520–537.

Farrington, R., Collins, L., Fisher, P., Danquah, A., & Sergeant, J. (2019). Clinical Debrief: learning and well-being together. *Clinical Teacher*, *16*(4), 329–334. https://doi.org/10.1111/tct.13055

Fegran, L., ten Ham-Baloyi, W., Fossum, M., Hovland, O. J., Naidoo, J. R., van Rooyen, D., Sejersted, E., & Robstad, N. (2023a). Simulation debriefing as part of simulation for clinical teaching and learning in nursing education: A scoping review. *Nursing Open*, *10*(3), 1217–1233. https://doi.org/10.1002/nop2.1426

Fegran, L., ten Ham-Baloyi, W., Fossum, M., Hovland, O. J., Naidoo, J. R., van Rooyen, D., Sejersted, E., & Robstad, N. (2023b). Simulation debriefing as part of simulation for clinical teaching and learning in nursing education: A scoping review. *Nursing Open*, *10*(3), 1217–1233. https://doi.org/10.1002/nop2.1426

Gray, J. R., & Grove, S. K. (2013). The Practice of Nursing Research: Appraisal, Synthesis, and Generation of Evidence – Seventh editionThe Practice of Nursing Research: Appraisal, Synthesis, and Generation of Evidence – Seventh edition. *Nursing Standard*, *27*(31), 30–30. https://doi.org/10.7748/ns2013.04.27.31.30.b1488

Guerrero, J. G., Tungpalan-Castro, G. M., & Pingue-Raguini, M. (2022). Impact of simulation debriefing structure on knowledge and skill acquisition for postgraduate critical care nursing students: three-phase vs. multiphase. *BMC Nursing*, *21*(1), 1–9. https://doi.org/10.1186/s12912-022-01100-z

Hensel, D., & Billings, D. M. (2020). Strategies to Teach the National Council of State Boards of Nursing Clinical Judgment Model. *Nurse Educator*, *45*(3), 128–132. https://doi.org/10.1097/NNE.0000000000000773

Høegh-Larsen, A. M., Gonzalez, M. T., Reierson, I. Å., Husebø, S. I. E., Hofoss, D., & Ravik, M. (2023). Nursing students' clinical judgment skills in simulation and clinical placement: a comparison of student self-assessment and evaluator assessment. *BMC Nursing*, *22*(1), 1–10. https://doi.org/10.1186/s12912-023-01220-0

Husebø, S. E., Reierson, I. Å., Hansen, A., & Solli, H. (2024). Post-simulation debriefing as a stepping stone to self-reflection and increased awareness — a qualitative study. *Advances in Simulation*, *9*(1), 1–12. https://doi.org/10.1186/s41077-024-00306-2

Ibrahim, A. F., & Aly, A. A. (2018). Clinical judgment among nursing interns. *Clinical Nursing Studies*, *6*(3), 19. https://doi.org/10.5430/cns.v6n3p19

Ided, W. H. O. P. (2014). The TIDieR (Template for Intervention Description and Replication). *Bmj*, 348.

Jensen, R. (2013). Clinical reasoning during simulation: Comparison of student and faculty ratings. *Nurse Education in Practice*, *13*(1), 23–28. https://doi.org/10.1016/j.nepr.2012.07.001

Jessee, M. A., & Tanner, C. A. (2016). Pursuing improvement in clinical reasoning: Development of the clinical coaching interactions inventory. *Journal of Nursing Education*, *55*(9), 495–504. https://doi.org/10.3928/01484834-20160816-03

Johnston, S. (2019). *An Evaluation of Simulation Debriefings on Student Nurses ' Perceptions of Clinical Reasoning and Learning Transfer : A Mixed Abstract :* 1–10. https://doi.org/10.1515/ijnes-2018-0045

Kavanagh, J. M., & Szweda, C. (2017). A crisis in competency: The strategic and ethical imperative to assessing new graduate nurses' clinical reasoning. *Nursing Education Perspectives*, *38*(2), 57–62. https://doi.org/10.1097/01.NEP.0000000000000112

Kawase, Y., Takahashi, S., Okayasu, M., Hirai, Y., & Matsumoto, I. (2024). Effectiveness of a Simulation-Based Education Program to Improve Novice Nurses' Clinical Judgment Skills. *Cureus*, *16*(6). https://doi.org/10.7759/cureus.61685

Kennedy, J. A., Laskowski, P. S., & Breyman, B. (2023). Clinical judgment in new nurse graduates: identifying the gaps. *International Journal of Nursing Education Scholarship*, *20*(1), 1–8. https://doi.org/10.1515/ijnes-2022-0112

Khan, M. H., Yaqoob, A., Sarwar, H., & Khan, S. (2021). The Impact of Standard in-Patients Exposure on Clinical Judgement among Undergraduate Nursing Students at SNC Lahore. *Pakistan Journal of Medical and Health Sciences*, *15*(11), 3109–3111. https://doi.org/10.53350/pjmhs2115113109

Kim, S., & Son, Y. (2022). Effects of Debriefing on Motivation and Reflective Thinking of Nursing Students during In-School Practicum Using a Flipped Learning Model. *Healthcare (Switzerland)*, *10*(12). https://doi.org/10.3390/healthcare10122552

Lasater, K. (2007). Clinical judgment development: Using simulation to create an assessment rubric. *Journal of Nursing Education*, *46*(11), 496–503. https://doi.org/10.3928/01484834-20071101-04

Lavoie, P., Pepin, J., & Cossette, S. (2015). Development of a post-simulation debriefing intervention to prepare nurses and nursing students to care for deteriorating patients. *Nurse Education in Practice*, *15*(3), 181–191. https://doi.org/10.1016/j.nepr.2015.01.006

Lavoie, P., Pepin, J., & Cossette, S. (2017a). Contribution of a reflective debriefing to nursing students' clinical judgment in patient deterioration simulations: A mixed-methods study. *Nurse Education Today*, *50*, 51–56. https://doi.org/10.1016/j.nedt.2016.12.002

Lavoie, P., Pepin, J., & Cossette, S. (2017b). Contribution of a reflective debriefing to nursing students' clinical judgment in patient deterioration simulations: A mixed-methods study. *Nurse Education Today*, *50*, 51–56. https://doi.org/10.1016/j.nedt.2016.12.002

Lavoie, P., Pepin, J., Cossette, S., & Clarke, S. P. (2019). Debriefing approaches for high-fidelity simulations and outcomes related to clinical judgment in baccalaureate nursing studentsLavoie, P., Pepin, J., Cossette, S., & Clarke, S. P. (2019). Debriefing approaches for high-fidelity simulations and outcomes re. *Collegian*, *26*(5), 514–521. https://doi.org/10.1016/j.colegn.2019.01.001

Lee, J. H., Lee, H., Kim, S., Choi, M., Ko, I. S., Bae, J. Y., & Kim, S. H. (2020). Debriefing methods and learning outcomes in simulation nursing education: A systematic review and meta-analysis. *Nurse Education Today*, *87*(April 2019), 104345. https://doi.org/10.1016/j.nedt.2020.104345

Levett-Jones, T., & Lapkin, S. (2014a). A systematic review of the effectiveness of simulation debriefing in health professional education. *Nurse Education Today*, *34*(6), e58–e63. https://doi.org/10.1016/j.nedt.2013.09.020

Levett-Jones, T., & Lapkin, S. (2014b). A systematic review of the effectiveness of simulation debriefing in health professional education. *Nurse Education Today*, *34*(6), e58–e63. https://doi.org/10.1016/j.nedt.2013.09.020

Lusk, J. M., & Fater, K. (2013). Postsimulation debriefing to maximize clinical judgment development. *Nurse Educator*, *38*(1), 16–19. https://doi.org/10.1097/NNE.0b013e318276df8b

Maestre, J. M., & Rudolph, J. W. (2015a). Theories and Styles of Debriefing: the Good Judgment Method as a Tool for Formative Assessment in Healthcare. *Revista Española de Cardiología (English Edition)*, *68*(4), 282–285. https://doi.org/10.1016/j.rec.2014.05.018

Maestre, J. M., & Rudolph, J. W. (2015b). Theories and Styles of Debriefing: the Good Judgment Method as a Tool for Formative Assessment in Healthcare. *Revista Española de Cardiología (English Edition)*, *68*(4), 282–285. https://doi.org/10.1016/j.rec.2014.05.018

Manetti, W. (2018). Evaluating the Clinical Judgment of Prelicensure Nursing Students in the Clinical Setting. *Nurse Educator*, *43*(5), 272–276. https://doi.org/10.1097/NNE.0000000000000489

Manetti, W. (2019). Sound clinical judgment in nursing: A concept analysis. *Nursing Forum*, *54*(1), 102–110. https://doi.org/10.1111/nuf.12303

Mariani, B., Cantrell, M. A., Meakim, C., Prieto, P., & Dreifuerst, K. T. (2013). Structured Debriefing and Students' Clinical Judgment Abilities in Simulation. *Clinical Simulation in Nursing*, *9*(5), e147–e155. https://doi.org/10.1016/j.ecns.2011.11.009

McCabe, D. E., Gilmartin, M. J., & Goldsamt, L. A. (2016). Student self-confidence with clinical nursing competencies in a high-dose simulation clinical teaching model. *Journal of Nursing Education and Practice*, *6*(8). https://doi.org/10.5430/jnep.v6n8p52

Modic, M. B., & Schoessler, M. (2013). Tanner's model of clinical judgment, part 2. *Journal for Nurses in Professional Development*, *29*(6), 335–337. https://doi.org/10.1097/NND.0000000000000017

Morse, C. J. (2013). The effect of debriefing with good judgment on acute care nurse practitioner students' reflective ability and perspective transformation. *VILLANOVA UNIVERSITY UMI Number: 3552408, ProQuest LLC (2013)*, 288 p-288 p.

Nielsen, A., Lasater, K., & Stock, M. (2016). A framework to support preceptors' evaluation and development of new nurses' clinical judgment. *Nurse Education in Practice, 19*, 84–90. https://doi.org/10.1016/j.nepr.2016.03.012

Nunes, J. G. P., Amendoeira, J. J. P., da Cruz, D. de A. L. M., Lasater, K., Morais, S. C. R. V., & de Carvalho, E. C. (2020). Clinical judgment and diagnostic reasoning of nursing students in clinical simulation. *Revista Brasileira de Enfermagem, 73*(6), 1–6. https://doi.org/10.1590/0034-7167-2018-0878

Oh, H. K. (2016). Effects on nursing students' clinical judgment, communication, and skill performance following debriefing using a clinical judgment rubric. *International Journal of Bio-Science and Bio-Technology, 8*(1), 303–312. https://doi.org/10.14257/ijbsbt.2016.8.1.27

Okada, M., & Tomari, Y. (2017). Thinking Process of Nursing Students' Clinical Judgment in Pediatric Nursing Practicum. *Open Journal of Nursing, 07*(11), 1258–1273. https://doi.org/10.4236/ojn.2017.711091

Ostovar, S., Allahbakhshian, A., Gholizadeh, L., Dizaji, S. L., Sarbakhsh, P., & Ghahramanian, A. (2018). Comparison of the effects of debriefing methods on psychomotor skills, self-confidence, and satisfaction in novice nursing students: A quasi-experimental study. *Journal of Advanced Pharmaceutical Technology and Research, 9*(3), 65. https://doi.org/10.4103/japtr.JAPTR_291_18

Palaganas, J. C., Fey, M., & Simon, R. (2016). Structured debriefing in simulation-based education. *AACN Advanced Critical Care, 27*(1), 78–85. https://doi.org/10.4037/aacnacc2016328

Persico, L. (2017). A Comparison of Two Debriefing Methods on Clinical Reasoning Outcomes, Learner Satisfaction with Debriefing and Reflection, Clinical Learning and Clinical Reasoning, and Psychological Safety of Nurse Orientees in Simulation-Based Education. *Comparison of Two Debriefing Methods on Clinical Reasoning Outcomes, Learner Satisfaction with Debriefing & Reflection, Clinical Learning & Clinical Reasoning & Psychological Safety of Nurse Orientees in Simulation-Based Education*, 1.

Reed, S. J. (2015). Written debriefing: Evaluating the impact of the addition of a written component when debriefing simulations. *Nurse Education in Practice, 15*(6), 543–548. https://doi.org/10.1016/j.nepr.2015.07.011

Rudolph, J. W., Simon, R., Rivard, P., Dufresne, R. L., & Raemer, D. B. (2007). Debriefing with Good Judgment: Combining Rigorous Feedback with Genuine Inquiry. *Anesthesiology Clinics, 25*(2), 361–376. https://doi.org/10.1016/j.anclin.2007.03.007

Sawyer, T., Eppich, W., Brett-Fleegler, M., Grant, V., & Cheng, A. (2016). More Than One Way to Debrief: A Critical Review of Healthcare Simulation Debriefing Methods. *Simulation in Healthcare, 11*(3), 209–217. https://doi.org/10.1097/SIH.0000000000000148

Shaub, K. Z. (2019). The Effect of Structured Debriefing on Prelicensure Nursing Students ' Clinical Judgment Development. *Nursing (Graduate) Student Scholarship.*

Shea, K. L. (2015). The effect of simulation with debriefing for meaningful learning in courses of nursing theory and practicum on student knowledge and perception of instruction. *The University of San Francisco USF Scholarship: A Digital Repository @ Gleeson Library | Geschke Center, Doctoral Dissertations. 299.*

Sultan, B., Dhamani, K., Ishtiaq, M., & Huda, S. (2024). *Effects of Structure Debriefing on Procedural Skills and Satisfaction of Nursing Students in Low Fidelity Context: A Pilot Study*. Atlantis Press International BV. https://doi.org/10.2991/978-94-6463-248-4_21

Sultan, B., Victor, G., & Begum Gul, R. (2024). Effect of Unfolding Case Studies on Critical Thinking Dispositions and Academic Performance of Undergraduate Nursing Students. *Annals of King Edward Medical University*, *29*(Spl3), 268–275. https://doi.org/10.21649/akemu.v29ispl3.5594

Sultan, B., Victor, G., Naeem, F., & Gul, H. (2024). Effects of Online Unfolding Case Studies on Clinical Reasoning and Academic Performance of Undergraduate Nursing Students. *Nursing Education Perspectives*, *00*(0), 1–3. https://doi.org/10.1097/01.nep.0000000000001244

Tanner, C. A. (2006). Thinking Like a Nurse : A Research-Based Model of Clinical Judgment in Nursing. *Journal of Nursing Education*, *45*(July 2006), 204–211. https://doi.org/10.3928/01484834-20060601-04

Van Graan, A. C., Williams, M. J. S., & Koen, M. P. (2016). Professional nurses' understanding of clinical judgement: A contextual inquiry. *Health SA Gesondheid*, *21*, 280–293. https://doi.org/10.1016/j.hsag.2016.04.001

Van Vliet, P., Hunter, S. M., Donaldson, C., & Pomeroy, V. (2016). Using the TIDieR checklist to standardize the description of a functional strength training intervention for the upper limb after stroke. *Journal of Neurologic Physical Therapy*, *40*(3), 203–208. https://doi.org/10.1097/NPT.0000000000000133

Victor-Chmil, J. (2013). Critical thinking versus clinical reasoning versus clinical judgment: Differential diagnosis. *Nurse Educator*, *38*(1), 34–36. https://doi.org/10.1097/NNE.0b013e318276dfbe

Vinícius, J., Felix, C., Caravaca-morera, J. A., & Bortolato-major, C. (2019). *Debriefing evaluation in nursing clinical simulation : a cross-sectional study*. *72*(3), 788–794.

Wallace, D. R., & Gill, J. M. (2019). The value of simulation debriefing in launching reduced anxiety and improved self-confidence in the clinical setting for accelerated baccalaureate nursing students. *Journal of Nursing Education and Practice*, *9*(7), 31. https://doi.org/10.5430/jnep.v9n7p31

Weaver, A. (2015). The Effect of a model demonstration during debriefing on students' clinical judgment, self-confidence, and satisfaction during a simulated learning experience. *Clinical Simulation in Nursing*, *11*(1), 20–26. https://doi.org/10.1016/j.ecns.2014.10.009

Yang, F., Wang, Y., Yang, C., Zhou, M. H., Shu, J., Fu, B., & Hu, H. (2019). Improving clinical judgment by simulation: A randomized trial and validation of the Lasater clinical judgment rubric in Chinese. *BMC Medical Education*, *19*(1), 1–6. https://doi.org/10.1186/s12909-019-1454-9

Yun, J.-A., & Kang, I.-S. (2022). The Effect of the Debriefing Method of Simulation Nursing Practice Education: A Literature Review. *Journal of Pharmacy and Nursing*, *2*(1), 1–11.

Zigmont, J. J., Kappus, L. J., & Sudikoff, S. N. (2011). The 3D Model of Debriefing: Defusing, Discovering, and Deepening. *Seminars in Perinatology*, *35*(2), 52–58. https://doi.org/10.1053/j.semperi.2011.01.003

Publisher: Eliva Press Global Ltd

Email: info@elivapress.com

www.ingramcontent.com/pod-product-compliance
Lightning Source LLC
LaVergne TN
LVHW022324200926
848481LV00004B/1426
9789999342070